Doctors Without Boredom

Dr. Barbara Newman

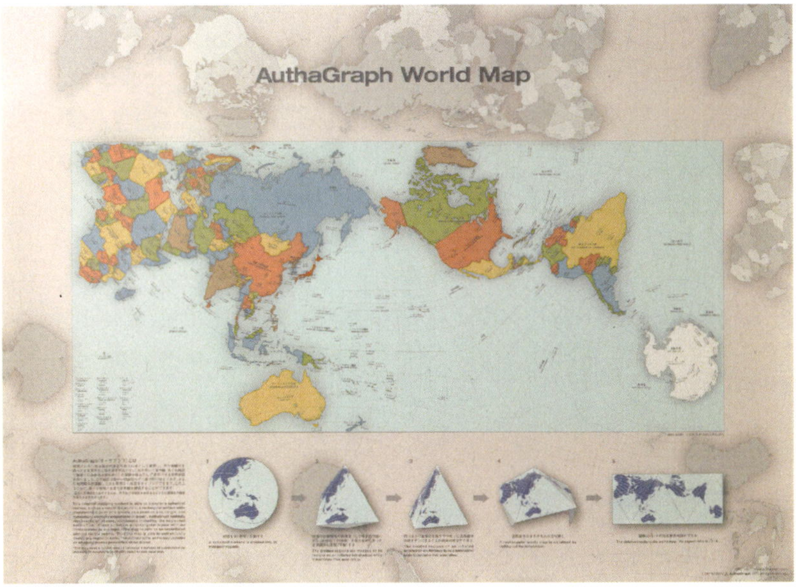

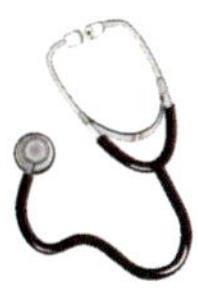

ISBN: 9798295418945

Dedication

To my father and mother, Leonard and Julia Newman, who inspired and supported me throughout their lives; and to my older sister Katy, who forged a path I proudly followed.

Acknowledgments

I benefited from the wisdom, experience, and sensitivity of the physicians, nurses, technical staff, and local healers with whom I have collaborated.

I want to honor the patients of Angola, Sudan, India, Mexico, Haiti, Alaska, South Dakota, and rural California, along with their families. Despite the scarcity of medications and materials and the lack of access to modern technologies or local care, they showed great resilience and humanity.

The organizations Lalmba and Doctors Without Borders/Médecins Sans Frontières (MSF) were instrumental in giving me and doctors like me opportunities to share our skills and knowledge.

I am deeply indebted to the many women who have courageously shared with me over the past 20 years their painful experiences of FGM (female genital mutilation). I am proud to have helped them obtain asylum in the United States through my medical examinations, published writings, court testimony, and speaking engagements.

My spoken word coaches at The Marsh Theatre in San Francisco enabled me to describe my work in accessible, entertaining ways.

I also wish to acknowledge the compassionate assistance of Attorney Paul Harris as well as my designer/editor Joshua Harris.

Guerrillalaw Publishing
Tapdoctor division
20 Quickstep Lane #1
San Francisco, Ca 94115

Contact emails:
Tapdoctor45@gmail.com
Guerrillalaw@earthlink.net

Design and Layout
by Josh Harris

CONTENTS

Note: These stories were originally created as spoken word performances. In certain stories the stage directions appear (CAPITALIZED IN PARENTHESES).

At the End of the World

Everything we'd done...had failed. I'd had this young woman balance on her hands and knees on the bed, while I gently jiggled her very pregnant belly in an effort to get the baby's head out of the pelvis where it was stuck. I'd had her lie on her back, while I reached over her belly down to where I could feel the baby's head, through the skin, and tried to manually pull it up out of the pelvis. Then I tried an internal approach, reaching into the vagina and through the uterine opening, which had stretched to its fullest extent, until I could feel the baby's head with my fingers. I gingerly pushed it up, trying to free it from the pelvic brim.

I was lucky to be working with a smart, experienced Haitian nurse, Kolet, in this small medical clinic in rural Haiti. She was the one who'd placed a catheter to make sure a full bladder wasn't in the baby's way; and started an IV infusion to prevent the mother's dehydration. I'd added a dose of antibiotics, in case there was an infection lurking somewhere. Then we repeated my maneuvers, but nothing changed. The baby's head remained stuck at the pelvis.

Let's talk about the pelvis. It's a bony girdle which encircles our bodies at about this level. Women have them, men have them, all mammals have a pelvis, and even most vertebrates. In the human female, one of its functions is to protect the reproductive organs and a growing fetus, if there is one, from injury. But when the fetus grows large enough to be born, the pelvis can become a formidable obstacle.

If this is your pelvis, the bone at the front is called the pubic bone. If you're not too squeamish, you can reach down and feel it through your clothes right now - it's below the waist and above the pubic area, it's hard (being a bone), and it's just under the skin. It actually is made up of two bones, the right pubic bone and the left pubic bone, joined by a thick wedge of cartilage. It's this structure under which the baby must dive, head first, to get into the birth canal and get born. If the baby's head is too big to fit under this barrier, or if the head is in the wrong position, extended back, instead of flexed forward, it can get stuck up against the pubic bone.

In our case, even though her uterus was open, and was contracting strongly enough to squeeze the baby out, the baby was stuck. This is called an obstructed labor; it's an obstetric emergency, a surgical emergency, because the safest way to treat an obstructed labor is to perform a cesarian section -- a surgical delivery. The mother and baby needed to be in a hospital with an obstetrician, or a general surgeon, and an operating room.

This was when I discovered the reason behind the nickname of this village. Its real name was Les Irois; its nickname, "The End of the World." I'd been here for three weeks, but this was the day that I found out the following:

1) The nearest fully equipped hospital was four hours away on bad roads, or five hours away by sea.

2) There were only two vehicles in the village - the priest's car, which was broken down, and the truck belonging to the village's richest man, which was out of gas.

I also discovered that a telephone landline had never been extended to Les Irois, much less a cell phone tower. Only the priest had a small two-way radio. I could neither telephone for help, nor go for help, at least not by road.

So Kolet and I went down to the beach. It was a beautiful sight: a clear blue sky, white sand, the turquoise Caribbean, palm trees swaying in the breeze. When we got to the water's edge, I noticed the wind had picked up. The entire bay was covered with foam, and some of the waves looked at least seven or eight feet high.

We told the head fisherman our story. He shook his head,

"No no *Dokte*, the sea is rough - I don't dare even take my boat out to fish, much less transport a pregnant woman in labor."

"*Map vini ak ou;* I'll come with you, I'll take care of the woman."

"Oh? Then we lose you too?"

"The priest has a radio. Can't we get him to call the Coast Guard?"

"No no, *Dokte*, his little radio only connects him to other priests."

"Please, monsieur! This is a matter of life and death! I'll pay for any gasoline you use. And I'll get your boat repaired if it gets damaged."

"*Dokte*," pause, "if this mother and baby are going to live, it will be God's will. We must trust in the *Bon Dye*. No more talk of going out on this rough sea today."

As we walked back through the village, over unpaved streets lined with small houses painted in bright colors, dodging chickens and the occasional pig, I got in touch with my feelings. I was furious!! Furious with the baby for being so big, at the petite mother for having such a small pelvis, at the Haitian government for failing to provide basic healthcare to all its people, at the Haitian project director who didn't live in the town where the health project was located, like me and Kolet, but chose to live in a town two hours away - with electricity, paved roads and clean water, where he kept the Jeep and shortwave radio with him. He only came once a week to bring supplies and mail. I was most angry at myself for not thoroughly investigating the situation on the ground before signing up to work here for six months! Above all, I was furious that mothers and babies are still dying preventable deaths in childbirth, in situations like this, all over the world, in the 21st century!!

Back at the hospital, we checked on mother and baby. They were stable - no fever, high blood pressure or hemorrhage. I could hear the baby's heartbeat through the mother's abdomen: fast and steady. Most important, the protective bag of waters surrounding the baby was intact - it hadn't been torn or punctured."Kolet, *sa n'ap fe kunya-la*?" What are we going to do now?

"*Dokte*! *Famn saj-la*?"

Great idea! The traditional midwife! She'd delivered so many babies, She must have tricks up her sleeves I'd never even thought of! She came as soon as we sent for her.

"*Mesi pou vini madam.*" Here's a fresh pair of gloves.

"*Oh? No no; pa pou mwen.*" I don't need them. "*Mamam, Papa, Dokte, Enfmye: gade!*" Watch!

She proceeded to walk around the bed five or six times, clapping, snapping her fingers, and praying to the Vodou gods to protect this mother and guide the baby out into the world. She finished with a turn, then looked at all of us.

"*Pa pe. Tout pral fini byen.*" Don't worry, everything will turn out fine. Everything. *"Ta le!"* And she gives a wave goodbye.

"Wait! Kolet, is that all she's going to do?"

"*M pa konne Dokte...*" She gestures, shrugging her shoulders.

Leaving Kolet in charge, I stepped out onto the hospital porch. My heart was pounding. The midwife had been our last hope. This was no longer an interesting medical quandary, or a logistical problem to be solved; nor a story to recount to colleagues over a beer at some later date.

I. Didn't. Know. What. To. Do.

But I had to calm myself down if I was to be any help to anyone.

(SIT)

I emptied my head of all thoughts, and began to meditate.

(CLOSE EYES FOR TEN BEATS OF SILENCE, THEN OPEN THEM).

A conversation from three weeks ago had popped into my mind. The doctor I was replacing was briefing me on what to expect here in Les Irois; it didn't take him long, he'd only been here a month. When he brought out a couple of cold beers, I could tell he was dying to talk medicine. I listened as he described interesting cases he'd seen in his last year of residency, just before he came to Haiti. He was young, clean cut, smart, a little cocky, I thought - a newly minted boy doc trying to impress me with his medical knowledge. In particular, he wenton and on about a procedure I'd heard of but never seen; it was of historical interest, but no one did it any more. Turns out he'd observed another doc actually performing it just before he came to Haiti. I couldn't figure out why he was going on and on. I mean, he drew diagrams, he acted it out. I finally said to him, "You know, Bob, it'll be a cold day in July before I do that."

Never say that - never even think that.

But wait...REMEMBER the two halves of the pubic bone, joined by a piece of cartilage? Well, the procedure he was describing, called a pubic symphysiotomy is actually pretty simple. You just take a scalpel and cut completely through that cartilage. The two halves of the pubic bone then separate, giving the fetus more room to dive under them and into the birth canal; and get born. It turns out that before we had metal forceps, with which we pull babies out by their heads, or vacuum aspirators with which we suck them out by their scalps, and before cesarian section surgery had been perfected, pubic symphysiotomy was commonly used in cases of obstructed labor.

Speaking of which...Mother and baby were still stable, but she was tiring and dad looked scared. The priest came in saying he hadn't found a car for us, but he'd organized a group of his parishioners into a prayer circle in front of the clinic. A kid ran in from the beach with a message from the fisherman: clouds were coming in and the sea was rougher; a small girl arrived to inform us that the rich man had just left on his mule for the gas. This meant that in eight hours - four to get the gas, and four to drive to the hospital - the mother could be in that hospital having a cesarian section. Or she and the baby could both be dead. An obstructed labor is nothing to take lightly - sure mother and baby were stable now, but if the condition of one or the other deteriorated, things could go downhill in a hurry. Symphysiotomy was looking better and better to me.

I took Kolet aside and explained it to her.

"*Sa ou dl? Ouap coupe zo?* You're going to cut her bones to get the baby out? I've never heard of such a thing! Desole, *Dokte*, I can't help you with that. If I have anything to do with it and something goes wrong, the people here will kick me out of the village! Then how will I support my kids?"

"*Ok, kolet, Ok. M kompran.* I get it. But just let me ask you one question: in your training and experience, have you ever seen an obstructed labor where there was no surgeon available?" (I WAIT 3 BEATS). "Two times? What happened? What happened, Kolet?"

(LOOK DOWN, FOLD ARMS ACROSS CHEST)

"You know what happens, *Dokte*; the babies died, and then the mothers died."

(5 BEATS, WIPE AWAY TEAR, DEEP BREATH IN AND OUT. LOOK UP.)

"Ok *Dokte*, what do you need me to do?"

As I collected supplies, I listened to Kolet explaining the plan to the parents. I admired the way she described it simply and clearly, matter-of-factly. Both parents nodded.

I stood in front of the mother to be. Her knees were bent, her legs on either side of me. I injected local anesthetic just under the skin where I was going to cut. Kolet scrubbed the entire area with iodine, and we both put on sterile gloves. While she dabbed up drops of blood, I carefully cut through the skin, and down through the layer of fat underneath, until I could see the cartilage. Then I sawed downward, slowly and steadily; it had the consistency of hard licorice.

(3 BEATS.)

I sawed till I felt it give.

Now when young Dr. Bob had described it to me, in my mind's eye I saw the 2 halves of the bone spring apart.

(GESTURE)

But what really happened? They separated by about an inch. An inch.

I was stunned. Had this failed too? What on earth was I going to tell these parents? They were staring at me; all I heard was her crying and his praying. Kolet backed away from me into a corner of the room. I have never felt so alone in my life. I made myself look at both parents, directly in the eyes. There was no turning back. I prepared myself to tell them… The Truth.

(OPEN MOUTH. 3 BEATS, JERK BACKWARDS)

A sudden splash of fluid soaked my scrubs. I saw something moving - Oh my god, it was the baby's head pushing out! "Kolet!"

We sprang into delivery mode (GESTURES) and before I knew it, a big baby girl was lying in my arms, screaming at the top of her lungs. I was so surprised to see her there, I couldn't move. It was Kolet who clamped and cut the umbilical cord, took the baby from me, dried her off and wrapped her in warm blankets. I pulled myself together, delivered the placenta, and sewed up the cut I'd made in the skin over the cartilage.

As I changed into dry scrubs in the next room, I realized I was grinning and crying at the same time. So was the mother when I went back in. Kolet had washed her and gotten her into dry clothes. I hugged the mother and the baby in her arms.

Kolet and I looked at each other. I took her hands, she squeezed mine. "*Mesi ampil*, Kolet. You took a big risk to help me. I'll never forget it."

"I didn't do it for you *Dokte*, I did it for the baby. *M'te f'el pou bebe-a*"

Dad had gone out to spread the word and buy a feast of bread, cheese, mangos, bananas - and beer.

When he came back in, I hugged him. The priest and his prayer group crowded in as we sat around the bed and feasted, while the baby tried her hand at nursing. The last one to arrive was the midwife.

"You see *Dokte*, I told you everything would come out all right!"

Camels

I'm a doctor, riding in a battered pickup truck across the flat, arid landscape of Northern Sudan. With me in the pickup is a young Sudanese driver, Solomon. While he and I don't share a common language, a warm handshake at the start of our trip, and shared smiles over some of the sights we see, have helped us connect. The only other passenger in the truck is Harold - a chubby, fifty-ish, balding American man. When I was hired as the medical director of this project, he was hired as the administrator.

Looking around, the landscape resembles an unending vacant lot, not at all what I was expecting. I mean, where are the sand dunes, the desert animals, the pyramids, for god's sake? And the huge River Nile flows through this region, but there's no water in sight, not to my eye.

We pass a couple of one-story, concrete buildings, whose windows gape like empty eye sockets. The only signs of life are a couple of hawks circling overhead. Then I start to see bushes, with recently washed clothing spread on them to dry. A few children appear, playing with balls and sticks. These are not empty houses, nor abandoned villages. People live here! Solomon suddenly slows the truck, and then stops it altogether to allow a herd of camels to cross the two-lane highway in front of us. Harold continues sleeping, but I? I am transfixed! Camel after camel, at least thirty of them, ranging in color from white to beige to dark brown, undulate placidly across the narrow asphalt highway each one, it seems to me, takes a moment to crane its neck and look directly at us. Their eyelashes are so long! They're unruffled, placid. It's so peaceful, I feel like music should be playing. I watch till they're all out of sight.

Wow!! A moment earlier I'd been asking myself what I was doing here. What had I gotten myself into, signing up to practice medicine for eight months in the middle of the desert?!

Watching the camels, I realize they know exactly what they're doing here. I need to learn from them.

Antonio's Story

The landscape in northern Angola is flat. After the sun sets, it stays light for another two hours. It's so peaceful! Antonio and I used to sit outside on the hospital porch, drink tea, and talk, as we watched the birds fly away and listened as the crickets started chirping. Since he was 18 and had never been out of Angola, he had so many questions for me that I did most of the chatting. One day, on the spur of the moment, I said,

"Tell me about your life."

"*Voce quer ouvir a minha historia, Doutora*? You want to hear my story? Why? I'd rather hear another of your stories...About your family, your city, your hospital...You see, we don't really have a tradition of talking about ourselves - our stories are to make us laugh, or to explain why the world is the way it is. Our stories teach us how to live.

What? You want to know about my family? My village? How I became a nurse?

I see.

This will be hard for me *Doutora*. But since it's you who are asking, I will try.

You need to know, my stories aren't like your stories.

I was happy growing up in my small village. I had my parents, my brothers and sister, uncles and aunties, my school friends... it was a peaceful life. But as I grew older, I sensed that something was wrong, that something bad was going on outside our village.

The war came when I was about 12. Savimbi's rebels marched into our village. They surprised us at daylight. 20 or 30 men. They were so big. Each one had a big gun. And they looked so angry.

"Nobody move! Nobody!"

"You! You! You two over there! And you girls! All of you! Don't try to hide! And you boys! You too, come over here!"

I nearly fainted when he pointed at me

"Follow me!"

The man in charge chose about 20 of us kids, all 11 or 12, mostly boys.

They made us put our hands on top of our heads and herded us out of the village. (TURN HEAD) Father was standing there; he looked hard at me but never said a word. Mother was clutching the younger ones, tears pouring down her face. She also was silent.

Later I understood how powerless they were against these big men with guns. But at the time I couldn't understand why they didn't even try to save us.

The rebels circled around us, so no one could escape. They made us walk, no stopping. We were hot, tired, and scared to death.

If someone tripped, a soldier turned and pointed his gun; we quickly helped each other up. All day we went on (PUSH GRASS ASIDE WITH ARMS) through the long grass (DUCK DOWN) under trees whose branches had grown together. The only time we got any water was when we walked through a stream.

(SCOOP WITH BOTH HANDS) We scooped the water into our mouths without even stopping. We just peed into our clothes if we had to.

It was dark when we got to their camp. More soldiers came out to look at us.

"Nobody move!"

They started separating the girls from the boys. The boy next to me held onto his sister's hand.

"Please, sir, don't take my sister! Don't take her!"

The soldier just shot him in the head, *Doutora*! Right next to me! I knew then what I had to do. I had to live *boca feishada*.

They gave all the boys but me guns. Maybe because I was smaller...? I was so jealous! What 12 year old boy doesn't want a real gun? And every morning at breakfast the others got an extra cup of water and 2 white pills. They laughed and sang with the soldiers, around their campfire at night. I'd grown up with these boys. They'd changed: they had so much energy, they were so sure of themselves. They barely noticed me anymore.

I was assigned to live and work with the medics, because one of them had been killed in a firefight the week before. No guns or drugs for me. I learned to dig bullets out of bloody flesh, then clean and sew up the wounds. I learned to set broken arms using sticks and long vines, to make crutches out of branches. I learned what to do when they brought wounded in: first, stop the bleeding, then treat the pain, then figure out what else needed to be done.

And they taught me about medicines - this pill for fever, you drink this syrup for coughing, this is for vomiting. I learned to give shots - this injection is for convulsions, this one's for pain. I also learned to recognize when there was nothing more to be done - that was a different injection.

The older medics yelled at me when I made mistakes; when I did something right, they just grunted. But when no soldiers were around, they were kind to me. I lived for their smiles. I loved them - I had no one else to love.

I couldn't stand to think about my family; the sadness paralyzed me, I couldn't speak; I could hardly breathe.

The girls didn't get guns or drugs either, *Doutora*. Each day one soldier wasassigned to hunt small game, which the girls cooked. They gathered wild berries, greens, and nuts; they washed the clothes, cleaned up the garbage. They carried the heavy cooking pots when we broke camp.

And whenever a soldier grabbed one of them from around the women's campfire, they had to go with him. Then we'd hear their screams.

Sometimes they brought them to us, after - crying, bleeding, barely able to walk. We'd comfort them with our eyes, a touch on the shoulder; then, inside our medical tent, we'd gently clean them up, and sew them up as best we could. If one of them got pregnant, they'd just leave her behind the next time we moved camp. The soldiers said the babies would cry and give away our position.

That was my life for the next three years, *Doutora*, always afraid, always hungry, always on the move; taking care of the sick and wounded, carrying heavy packs of medicines and bandages, which the soldiers stole every time they marched into a village. I stopped wondering when it all would end, if it would ever end.

I must've been about 15 when one day a kid we didn't know ran into camp.

"Savimbi is dead! He's dead! He's dead! His bodyguard shot him! Savimbi is dead!! The war is over!"

Total silence in the camp. Then all of a sudden everyone started running around, grabbing their things. One of the medics hugged me.

"Get out! Now! Go home Antonio!"

I never saw him again. I grabbed some food and water and started walking with a few guys from my village. One of them knew what direction we should go in. I never saw any of the girls again - they'd been out gathering food when all this happened.

We walked west across Angola, toward the sea. We passed through burnt villages where dead bodies of villagers - men, women and children - were scattered on the ground. We heard no birds, no crickets; we saw no footprints.

When we came across other groups of walkers, we froze. There were so many rumors of groups of former rebels traveling around stealing food, raping, setting fires, that we were all scared to death of each other. At least one person in every group had a gun. Luckily as soon as one of us said a few words, someone in the other group recognized his dialect, and the guns were put away. That was one of the worst things about the war, *Dottora* - it took away our trust in each other

When we got to my village, it was gone. Everything burned to the ground. I stayed; the others went on. I had longed for this place for three long years. I couldn't just leave. I didn't see anyone. I thought it was empty, I sat down on the ground. Such loneliness...but then I saw this old man walking toward me.

"Tonio? Antonio?"

Uncle!

I thought he was the only one from my family still alive, but then my sister showed up. It wasn't hard for me to figure out what she had gone through. She rarely talked, and spent most of her time with the other women and girls. One night the three of us told our stories of the war to each other, around the fire. We talked for hours. But after that, we never spoke of it again.

Over the next few weeks and months people straggled back to the village in twos and threes. Most of us decided to stay, to rebuild. You'll like this *Doutora*: they chose me to be the village doctor! At age 15! Well, no one else knew how to take care of sick or injured people.

Doctors Without Borders came to our village about a year ago. They built a clinic and hired me as a nurse! They gave me a lot of training. I finally started to see how the human body is put together, how people get sick, how medicines help, how wounds heal. Then 3 months ago they sent me here, to work in this project.

So that's it *Doutora*. My life, my story. I have to go now."

For the next couple of weeks, even though he came to work every day, Antonio sort of disappeared. Even when our paths crossed, he never met my eyes, never spoke. I was so hurt - hurt? I was bereft! Friends are hard to come by in these isolated projects - I didn't know why I had lost this one. Then one day Mr. Gomes, the Angolan director of the project, pulled me aside.

He told me that since the war ended, people try not to ask ask someone a question if the answer will make him uncomfortable, or unhappy because sadness spreads to other people; everyone starts remembering. It makes everyone sad. He asked me,

"Please, *Doutora*, don't break this tradition."

Instant, endless remorse. I was so ashamed of my insensitivity. I dwelled on it. It became hard for me to eat or sleep.

Two or three weeks later Antonio and I were sewing up some deep cuts on a boy who'd fallen into a barbed wire fence. Antonio was on the right arm, I was working on the left leg. The kid was scared and in pain, shivering. To try to cheer him up, I made some kind of silly joke, no response. After two more stupid jokes, in Portuguese of course, he finally laughed. I started laughing with him.

When Antonio joined in our laughter, and looked me straight in the eyes, it felt like a boulder had just rolled off my heart...

Ra-Ra

I sat on the back of the motor scooter, lightly holding onto Pierre's waist. We were in rural Haiti, where I was doing medical work. He was giving me a ride to the next town, so I could make a phone call home. We're coworkers at an international NGO (charitable organization). The wind had evaporated our sweat on that humid day, and I was enjoying looking at the sparkling Caribbean on my left. On our right were small thatched houses surrounded by peanut fields, bananas, and mango trees; not a cloud in the sky.

Suddenly we passed an isolated thatch-roofed building - a house? store? - which was completely on fire. No one was around, and Pierre didn't comment on it, so neither did I.

Strange... About 10 minutes later, I noticed some movement up ahead. Gradually a group of men came into view As they got closer, I saw it was a large group. I heard a drum beating, and what sounded like chanting. Neither we nor they were moving very fast. I felt my heart in my chest; I was suddenly scared, sweating, gripping Pierre tightly now. I could hear their bare feet pounding on the dirt road.

What was going on? Hundreds of Black men running toward me? What were they going to do to me? I became aware of the smell of Pierre's sweat, his scratchy shirt; I saw that a number of the men were carrying torches. My mouth was dry; all the B movies I'd seen of hoards of "natives" descending on white colonists, raping, murdering - passed through my mind. The terror I felt was primal, not even at the level of conscious thought. I KNEW they were after me because I'm white. Visions of what they might do to me flashed before me.

I shouted inanely into Pierre's ear,

"*Yo fache ak mwen*? Are they mad at me?" It was all I could come up with in my far from perfect Kreyol. He looked at me, astonished. I continued,

"*Yo pa remen blanc-yo*? Do they hate Whites?"

Now he gave a short, harsh laugh.

"Despite all the things they've done to them, these uneducated country people still love the Whites. *Pa pe*, Barbara. *Yo konnelm. Yo pa oue ou. Se Ra-Ra*. Don't be afraid Barbara. They know me. They don't even see you.

It's just *Ra-Ra."*

True enough, they just passed around us.

The rest of the day was uneventful, peaceful. I later learned this was an annual ritual, with roots in Vodou, with colorfully dressed groups of young people, competing to be the flashiest, the most compelling, running through the streets.

Another lesson for white people: It's not always about YOU.

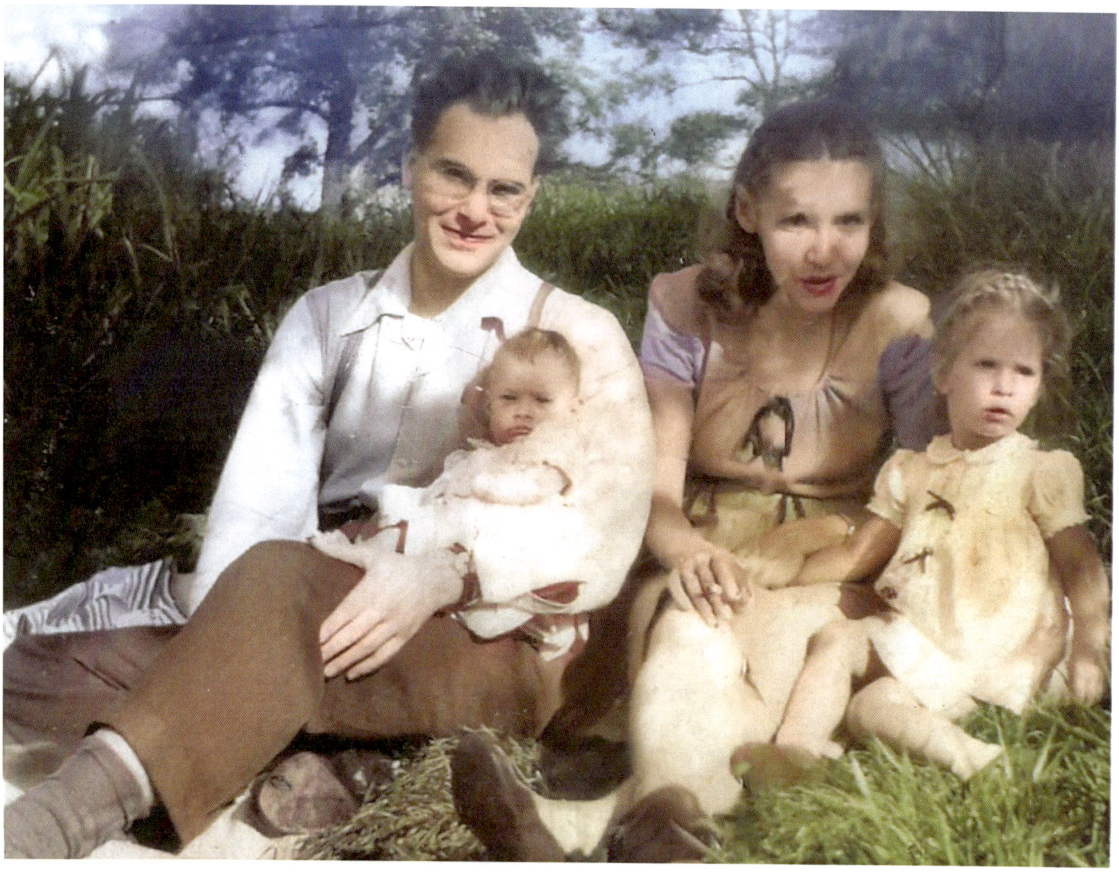

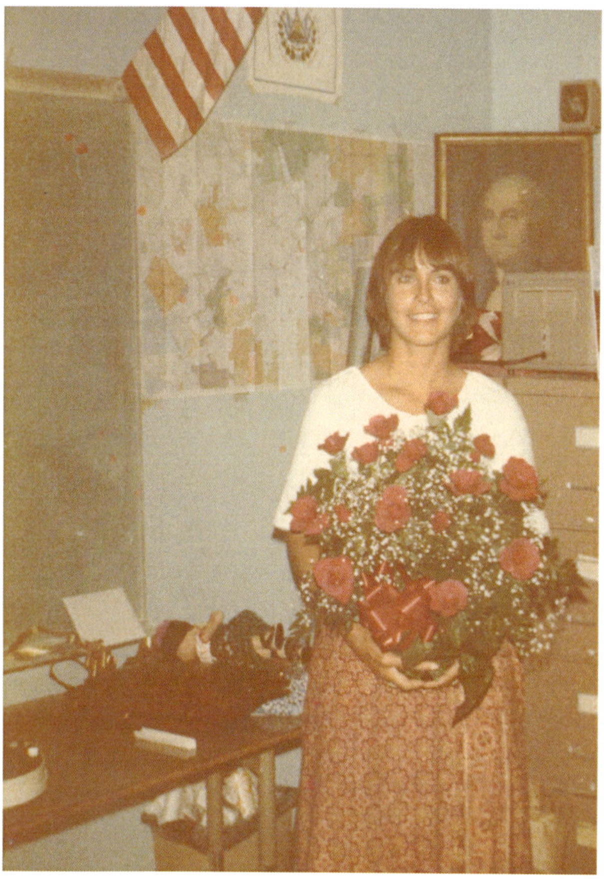

Parents Lenoard and Julia, baby Barbara and sister Katy. Los Angeles.1945

Teaching English as a Second Language. Los Angeles, California. 1979

After graduating UCLA Barbara became a belly dancer in New York. During 4 years she also performed in Puerto Rico, Las Vegas, and San Francisco. 1967

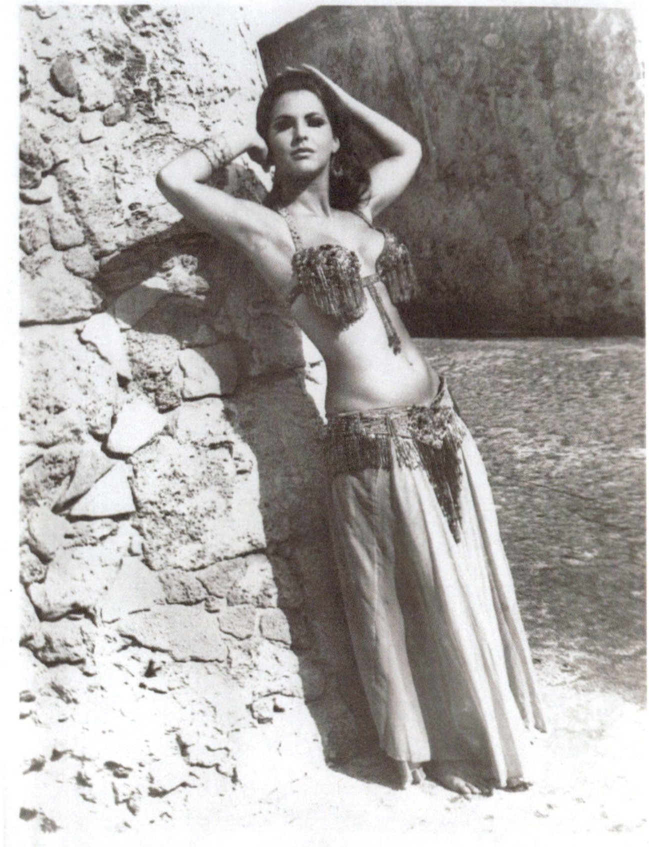

On vacation in Louisiana while getting both a M.D. and a Masters in Public Health at Tulane University Medical School. New Orleans. 1983

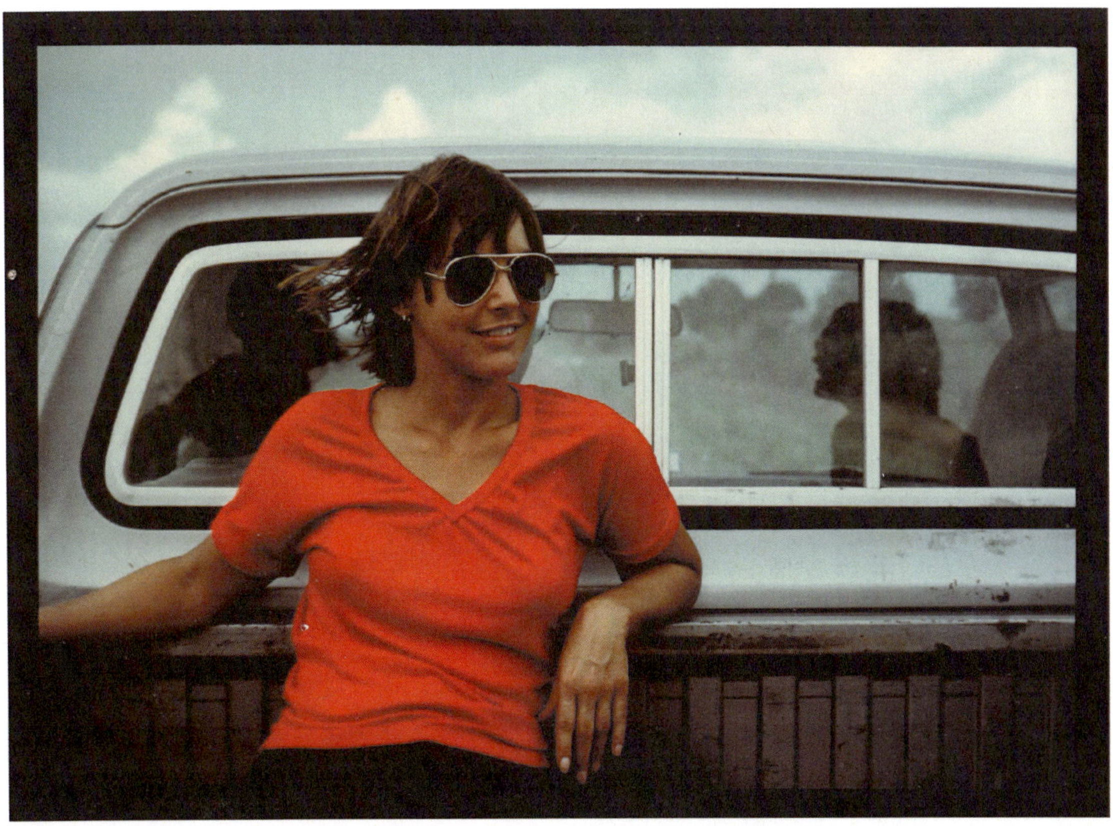

Trip Appalled Dr. Newman

'War Crimes' Cited in Salvador

By John O'Brien
Staff Writer

Among those who marched in protest to the entrance of Fort Benning Saturday was a physician who made no speeches but had a slew of things to say to the U.S. government about its foreign policy on El Salvador.

Dr. Barbara Newman's role in the march was to provide medical assistance to the 250 people who walked down Fort Benning Road to protest the training of Salvadoran soldiers at the post, but she was also one of about a half-dozen marchers who has actually been to the war-ravaged Central American country.

Dr. Newman, from New Orleans, was only in El Salvador for 10 days in March. She went to observe medical conditions in the country, and returned appalled.

"The lack of health care by the government is nothing short of murder," she says. "And that's in addition to the outright killing that's been going on since 1979."

But she carries with her a document that is more significant than her own observations. She says she was, after all, only in the country long enough to get a glimpse of the situation.

That document is a transcript of the testimony Dr. Charles Clements made to the House Subcommittee on Human Rights in March. In it he reveals the "war crimes" and the plight of U.S.-trained Salvadoran soldiers he witnessed while giving health care to peasants in the rural areas of El Salvador from March 1982 to March 1983.

See DR. NEWMAN, Page B-7

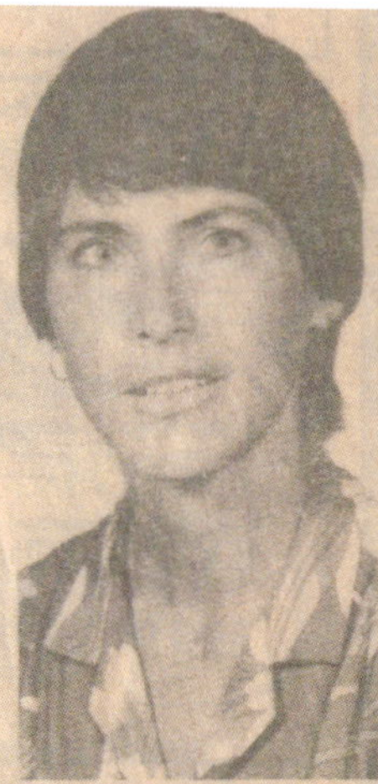

DR. NEWMAN

Fort Benning, protest after trip as a medical observer to El Salvador. 1982

Cheyenne River Reservation. South Dakota. 1989

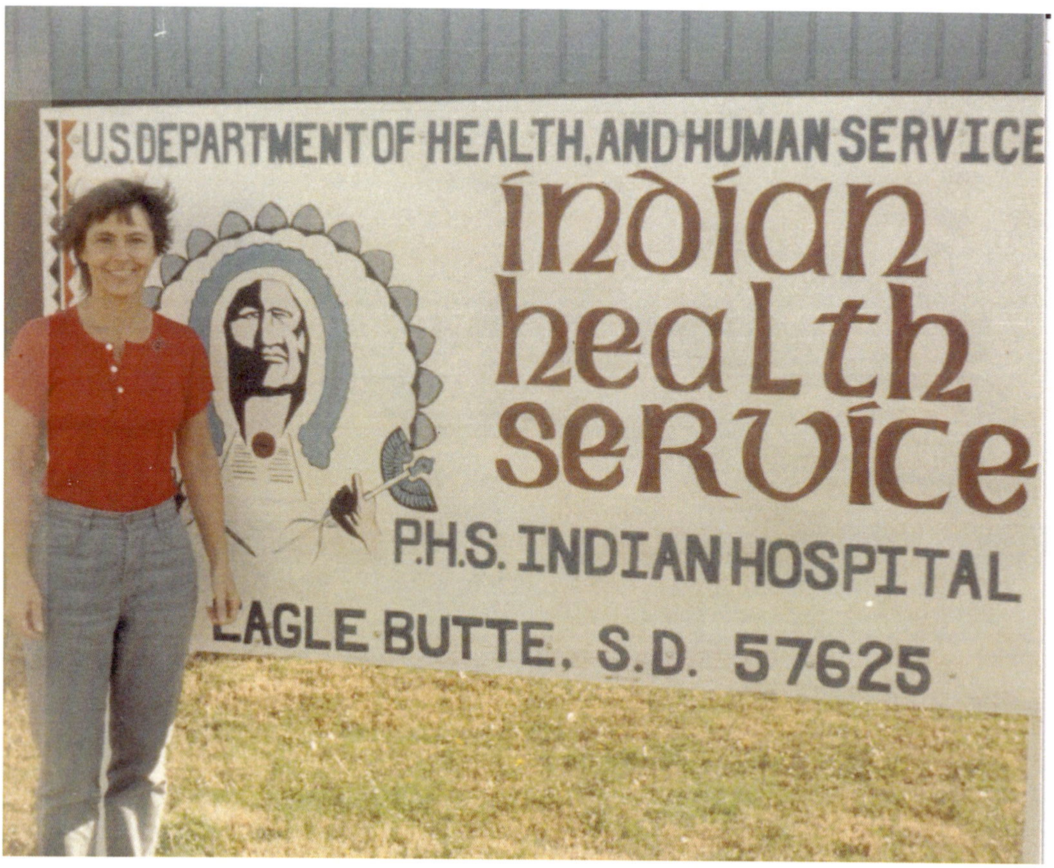

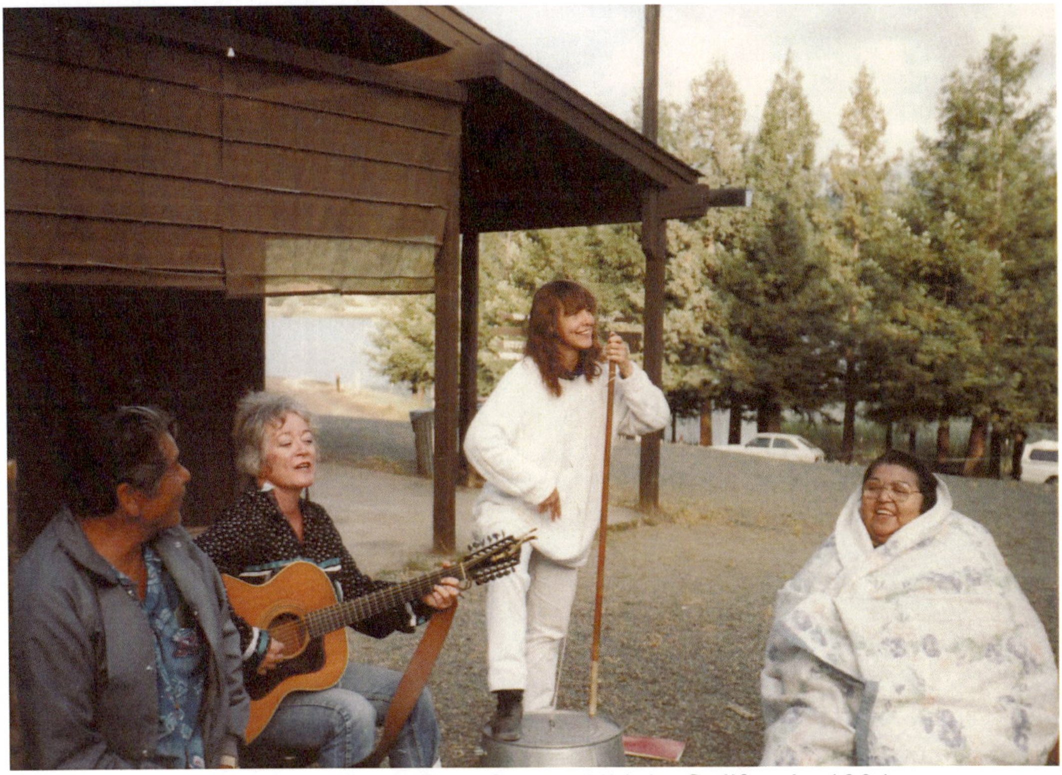

Diabetes Education Camp. Ukiah, California.1991

Campaign for Single Payer Prop 186, California. 1994

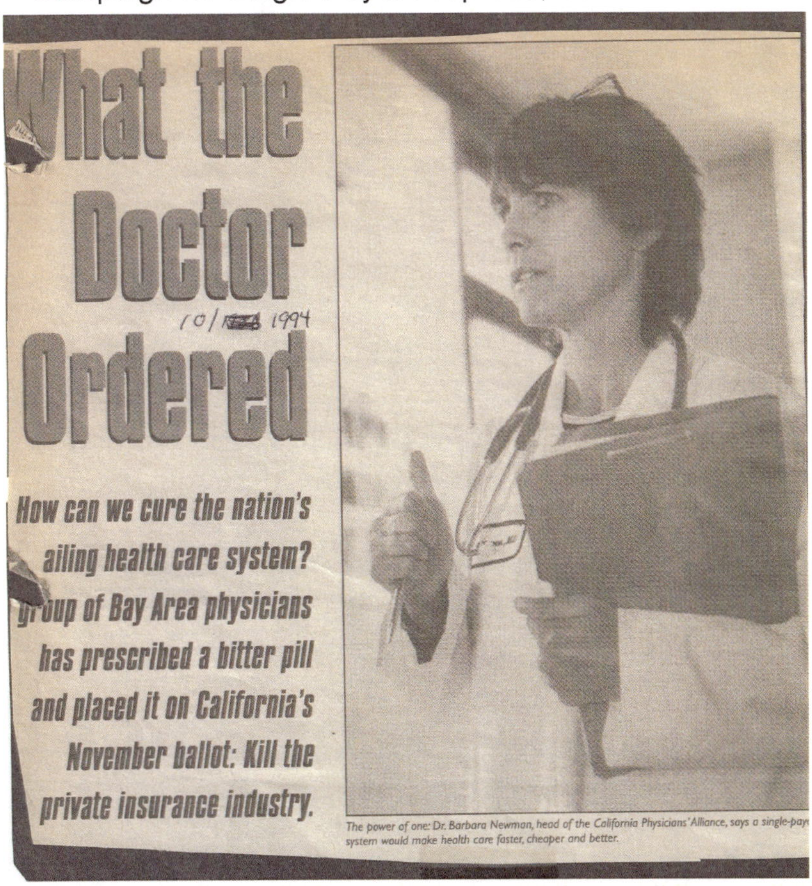

What the Doctor Ordered

10/ 1994

How can we cure the nation's ailing health care system? group of Bay Area physicians has prescribed a bitter pill and placed it on California's November ballot: Kill the private insurance industry.

The power of one: Dr. Barbara Newman, head of the California Physicians' Alliance, says a single-pay system would make health care faster, cheaper and better.

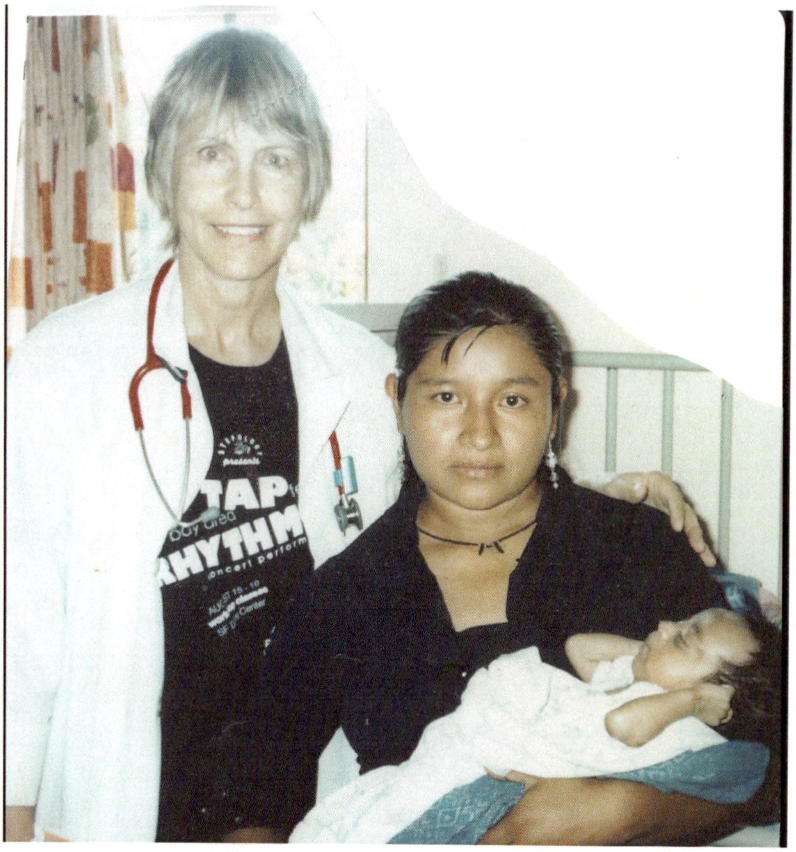

Delivered baby,
Chiapas, Mexico.
2000

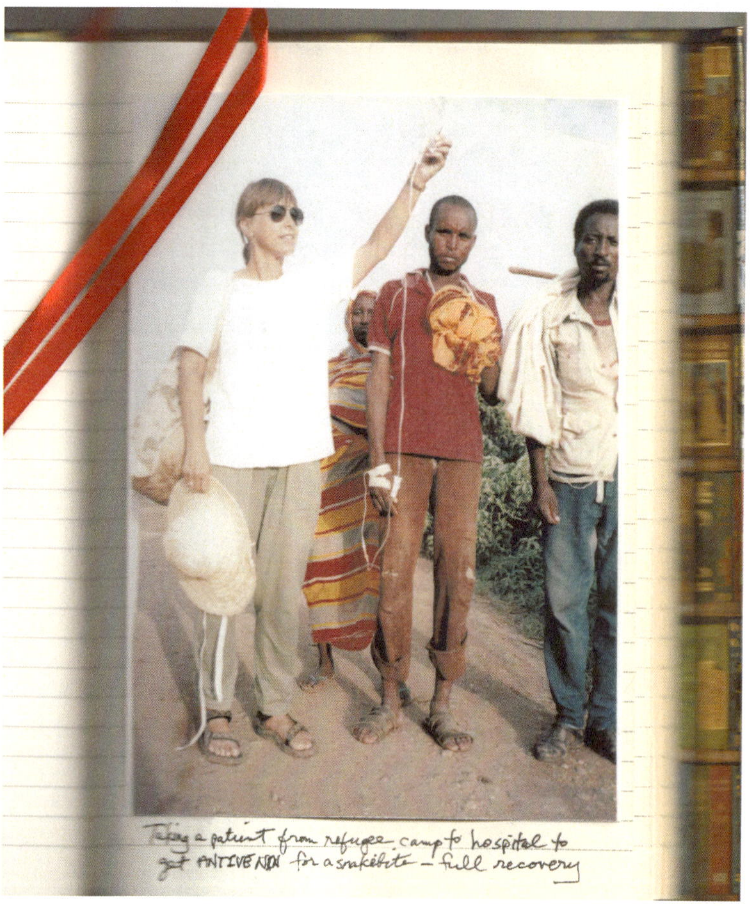
Taking a patient from refugee camp to hospital to
get ANTIVENOM for a snakebite – full recovery

Holding IV to treat
snakebite victim.
Sudan. 1995

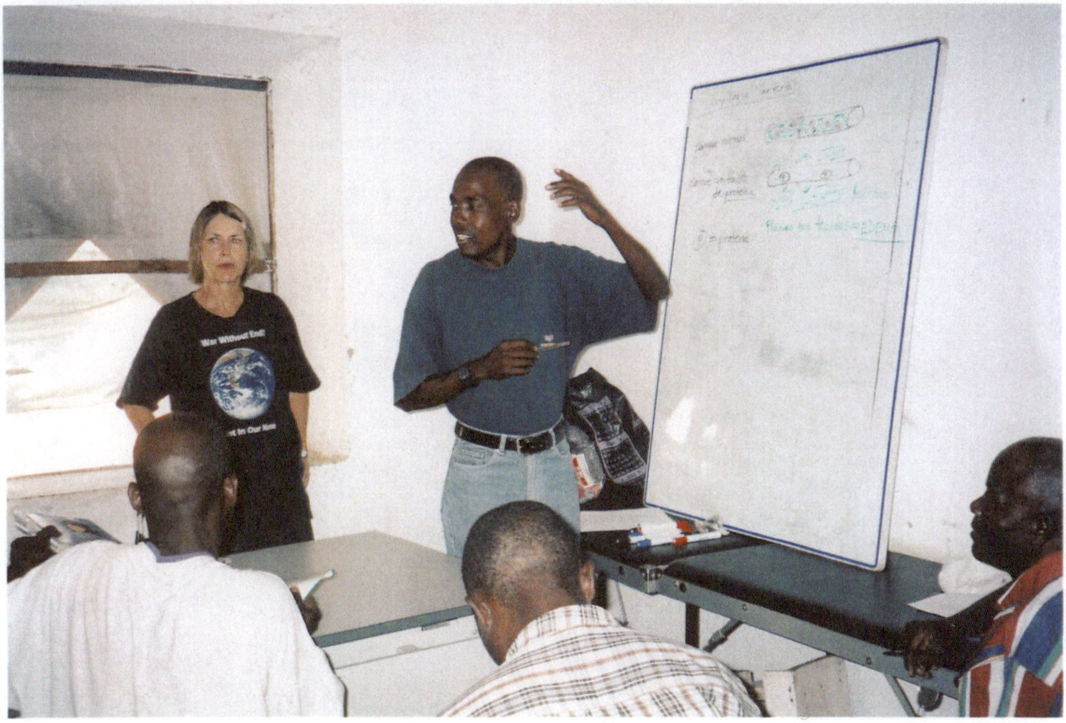

Teaching Ethiopian and Eritrean health workers in a refugee camp. Showak, Sudan. 1996

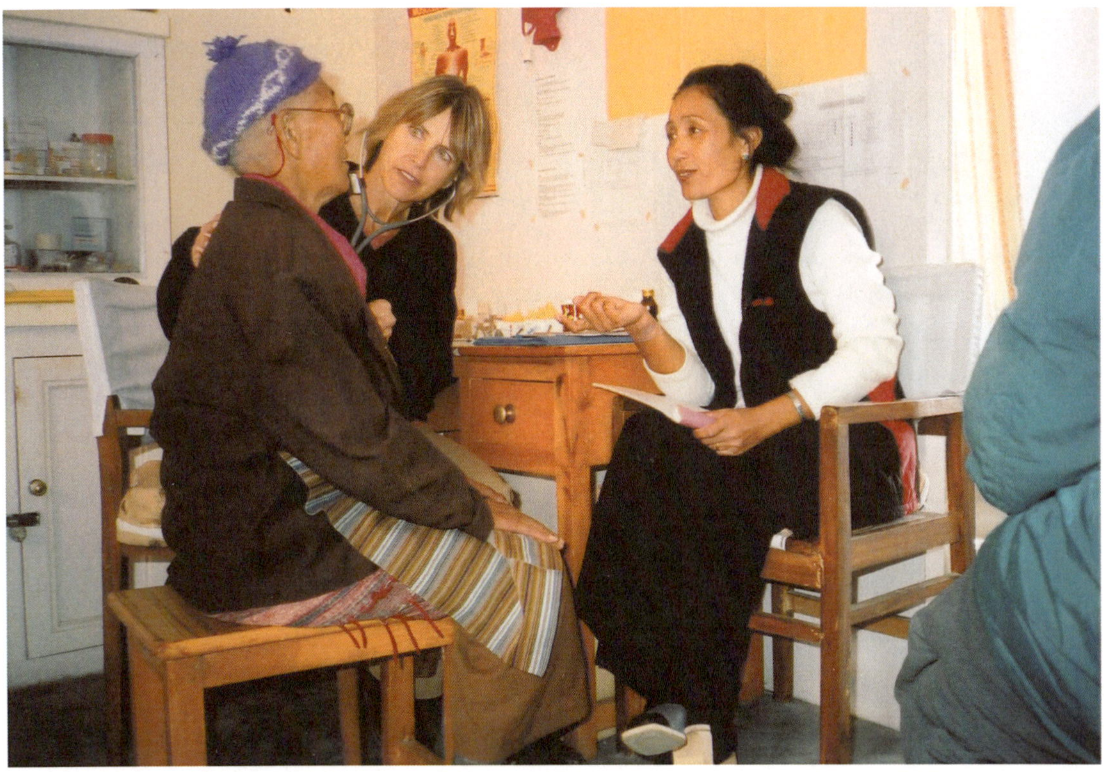

Delek Tibetan Hospital. Dharamsala, India. 2003

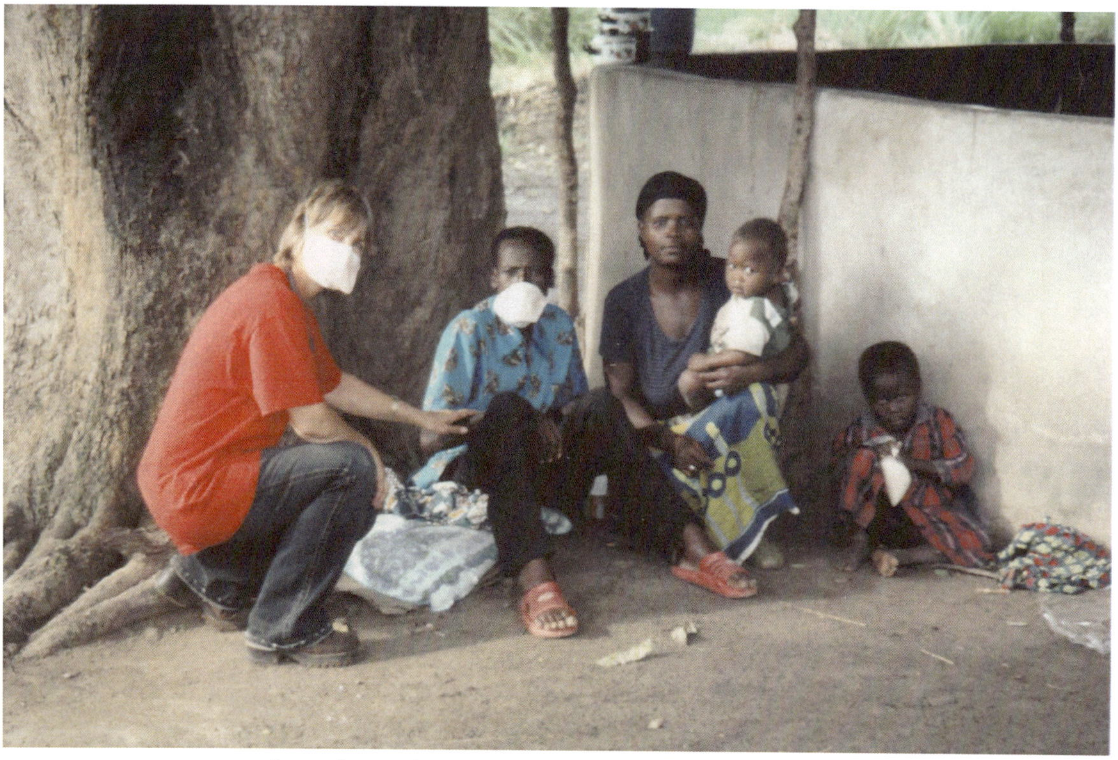

Creating a T.B. Clinic. Rural Angola. 2005

At home in St. Francis Square Co-op, San Francisco.

, Vol. 44 • No. 2 Election 3/19/2010

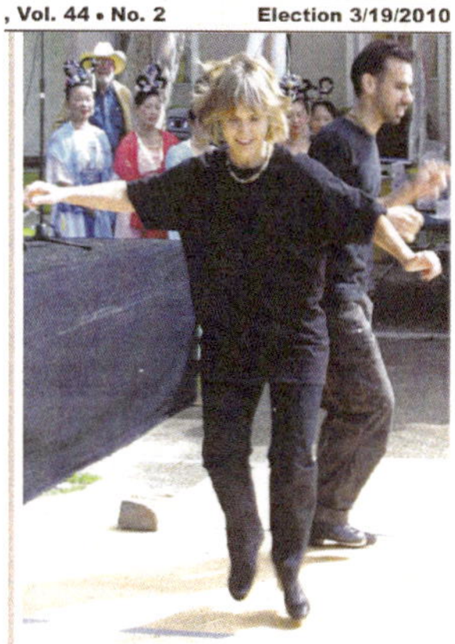

Barbara Newman tap-dancing at Square picnic

Our Own Doctor Without Borders

Photo & Story by Vicki Strang

Barbara Newman M.D. has volunteered to take her special skills in Emergency Medicine to help Haiti's earthquake victims. Stationed now about 150 miles outside of Port-au-Prince, she is part of a medical team assembled by Doctors Without Borders (Medecins sans Frontieres), the international medical relief organization that was awarded the Nobel Peace Prize a few years back.

This is not Barbara's first trip to Haiti. She worked there about 12 years ago, so she brings to this current assignment a slightly rusty knowledge of Creole and fluent French. On a prior stint with Doctors Without Borders she worked in Angola for several months. She expects to be back in the Square in two months.

Meanwhile, if you wish to make a contribution in support of Barbara's efforts, drop your check off at the Square office, payable to Doctors Without Borders. The staff of Circling the Square will make sure it gets to the medical team in Haiti. ■

With husband Paul Harris, San Francisco.

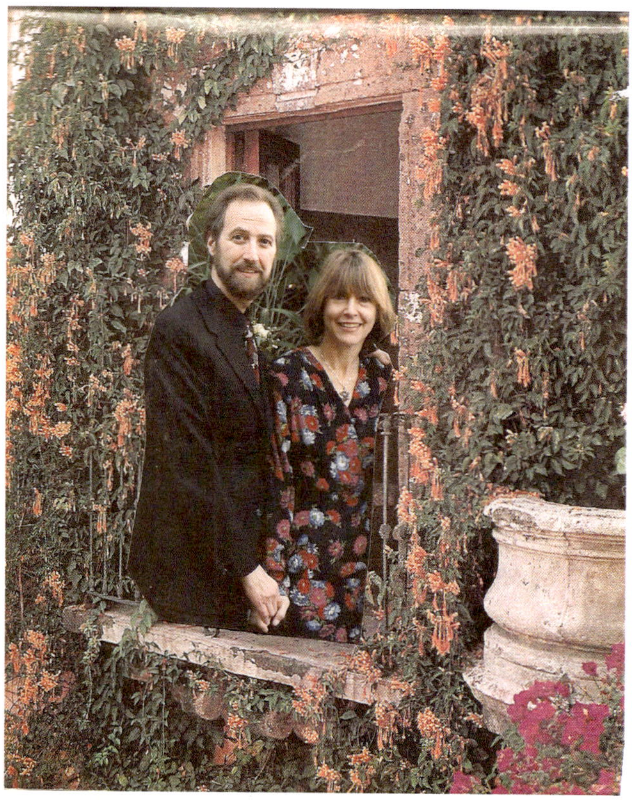

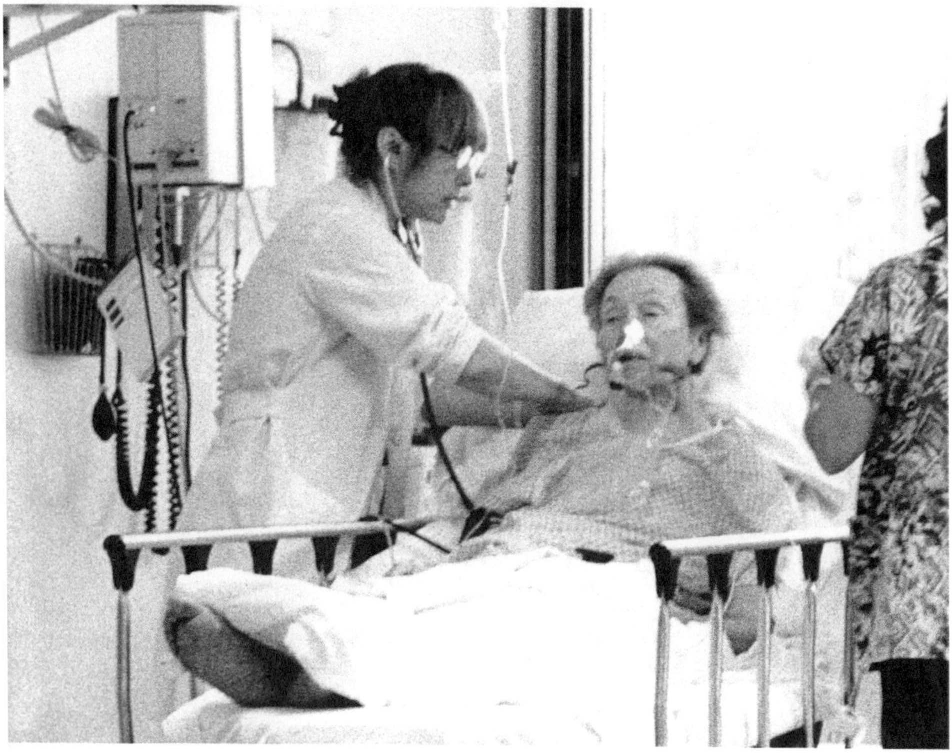

Emergency Room. Merced, California. 2011

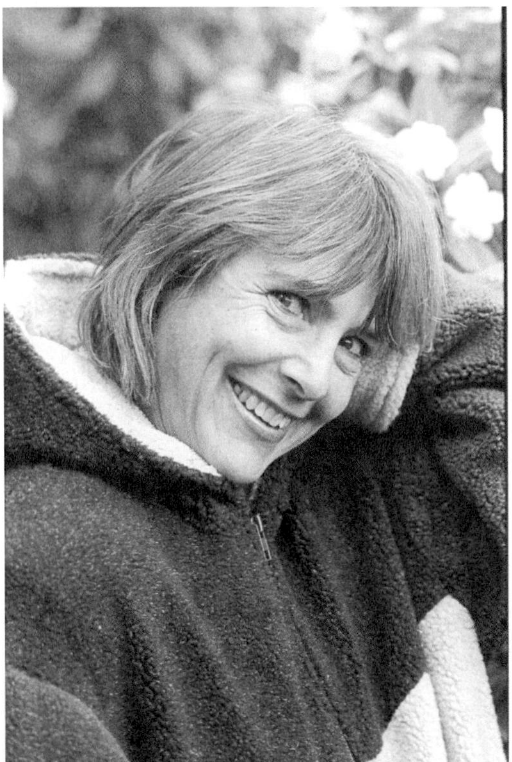

Marcos

I stared at the boy lying on the bed. He looked about 11 or 12, slender but sturdy. His dark eyes stared back at me. Tears streamed down his face. He was trembling all over, grimacing in pain. On the front of his dirty, oversized T-shirt was a large, fresh, red stain. I helped the nurse, Fernando, slip the shirt off over his head. Now we could see the gaping wound: about three inches long, just below his bellybutton, dripping dark red blood. As Fernando started an IV of saline solution, I put my stethoscope on the boy's belly: none of the usual growls or gurgles, just ominous silence. His heart was beating fast but steadily, both lungs were pumping air. A quick look at his arms and legs, chest, and face showed no other injuries. We carefully turned him up onto one side: no exit wound no injuries there.

"What's your name, sweetheart?"

"Marcos."

"Does it hurt a lot?"

"Yes."

I stroked his head as I spoke to him.

"We're going to give you some nice medicine to take the hurt away, but first Fernando will give you a shot."

He looked wildly at his mother. She nodded firmly. As soon as he got a dose of morphine, Marcos began to relax. I gently cleaned his wound, packed it with gauze, and wrapped a tight bandage around it to stop the bleeding. His breathing and pulse were starting to slow down and his blood pressure had not dropped. As the saline and antibiotics dripped in, we covered him with a light blanket. Then we also began to relax.

The whole thing had started around 5 pm as I was finishing dinner with my coworkers in the tent which served as our living quarters. Suddenly there was an earsplitting explosion, so loud it left us all temporarily deaf. I left the tent and ran through the village, up to our small hospital. *"Mina"* everyone was murmuring as I passed. We all knew that a sound like that could only mean one thing: a landmine left over from the civil war had been set off by someone driving or walking over it. It was my worst nightmare. As the only doctor in an isolated hospital in rural Angola, I worked with a wonderful crew of local nurses, but we had few resources.

I had fervently hoped that there would be no victims, but I'd found Marcos when I got to the hospital. Now I turned to Marcos' mother, who had been praying nonstop since she'd carried him into the clinic. She grasped my hand as she answered my questions, staring intently into my eyes. I could see her son's blood drying on her blouse.

"Yes, it was a landmine. Every day I tell him never to play outside our neighborhood unless he's on a road or a path we use. Every day!!

"But today the boys and girls were chasing each other in the grass alongside the road, and (COVER EYES WITH BOTH HANDS) he must've stepped on a mine. (ANGRY) The government was supposed to get rid of those terrible things, but it's been 4 years! They always forget about the poor people! (WIPE EYES) No, no one else was hurt, only my son. Please save him *Dottora*, please!"

I looked into her eyes and squeezed her hand. I had no words for her. We both knew the truth: her boy might die. Our biggest obstacle to getting this boy what he needed was the time of day: dusk. Night driving in rural Africa is notoriously dangerous: the highways are unlit, cars and trucks may be missing headlights or tail lights, wild animals cross the roads without warning, and, because of the threat of landmines, disabled vehicles are rarely moved off the road. So Doctors Without Borders has an ironclad rule: no night transports.

Marcos had been injured too late to be transported to the nearest well-equipped hospital (six hours away) until the next morning. And he needed to go. We had no surgeon. With such a deep wound and so much pain, the boy likely had fragments of shrapnel in his abdomen. Only a surgeon with an anesthetist to sedate Marcos could cut open his belly to remove the shrapnel and sew up any severed blood vessels or lacerated intestine. My job was clear: to keep him alive till 6 am. And all I had were IV solutions, morphine, and antibiotics.

I explained all this to Marcos' mother and Fernando. I watched his mother's face fall when I explained there could be no trip to the big hospital that night. She sat silently crying. I checked on the boy one last time. He was groggy but stable. He opened his eyes as I touched his hand and called his name, and even tried a wan smile in response to my thumbs up. His mother sat with her hand on his forehead. I touched her shoulder as I went out.

I walked back to the tent as night fell, passing through the villagers standing vigil. I didn't expect to sleep much. Sure enough, I was awakened around 3 am by the guard shaking my shoulder. I raced up to the hospital where I found Marcos hot to the touch, fitfully moaning, unconscious. His breathing was noisy and labored, his heart was racing. His BP had dropped to a dangerously low level. He was in shock. His abdomen was more swollen than when I had left. Fernando had turned both IVs wide open when he checked the blood pressure. I gave the boy a small dose of morphine, and set his mother to placing wet cloths all over his body to break his fever.

While Fernando prepared an extra antibiotic infusion, I went to our supply cupboard. After pulling nearly all our stock of IVs off the shelves, I found two bags of Hemacell solution as thick as blood, specifically used for shock. I grabbed one of them, along with the biggest IV tubing I could find, and ran back to the bedside. Marcos' fever had started to go down and he was calmer, but he still had noisy, rapid breathing and a swollen belly.

With Fernando supporting him in a sitting position, I lubricated his right nostril with ointment and gently threaded the IV tubing into it. When it reached the distance I'd estimated to his stomach, I attached a small syringe and pulled back. Nothing. I changed to a larger syringe for more suction and a watery, brownish fluid started flowing out. Fernando kept Marcos upright as I alternated, pulling and emptying the syringe. Over and over. After taking out about a liter, I saw that his belly was going down and his breathing was easier. Over the next hour, we slowly dripped half a bag of Hemacell into his veins and his BP gradually came up to normal.

But I was not leaving this kid's side until the van came to get him at 6 am. So I settled into one of the clinic chairs. Fernando disappeared briefly then reappeared, carrying two cups of hot tea with milk and sugar. Nothing had ever tasted so delicious.

Then followed the sweetest memory of my entire six months working in Angola. Seated in metal folding chairs, blankets wrapped around us, drinking sweet tea, we chatted quietly about our families. An anecdote about his youngest child's first steps was followed by my description of the first time I held my granddaughter in my arms and she nestled into me, holding tightly onto my finger. He asked me how my husband and I had met, and was charmed by the fact that we've known each other since Paul was 16 and I was 14. Fernando told me some of his wartime experiences, constantly on the run with his mother and brothers from raids by members of Savimbi's group, Unita, terrified all the time, nothing to eat but cress, his baby brother starving to death.

We checked on Marcos every half hour. He remained stable, sleeping. His mother had arranged herself on the floor beside his bed. Wrapped in blankets, she slept too.

Fernando woke me at a quarter to six. Our patient was stable, looking around. His mother was moistening his lips with a wet cloth. Fernando went with Marcos and his mother in the van, armed with Hemacell, antibiotics and morphine. He promised to call us on the satellite phone as soon as they arrived. I staggered home as the van drove off. I knew the nurses would go on.

TB Brothers

(STAND BEHIND CHAIR, HANDS ON THE CHAIRBACK.)

It was hot, humid, and so dark inside the large army tent where we slept. Through the curtains I could hear that the others were sleeping, some were snoring. Even our pet cat, *Princesa*, was snoring. Finally I gave up and tiptoed out of the tent and across the cement floor of the warehouse, trying not to wake anyone up.

You may be asking yourselves why we slept in a tent inside the warehouse. Well, when Doctors Without Borders rented this warehouse for their medical project near Malanje, Angola, they didn't realize that the warehouse already had a tenant. A colony of bats lived in the eaves of the warehouse, right over the sleeping area. Bats carry a lot of diseases. The tent was there to protect us from breathing the fine mist of batshit which wafted down from time to time.

From the steps of the warehouse...

(SIT)

...Wow!! I was blown away by the sheer number and brilliance of the stars. It was very peaceful. I heard a dog barking somewhere far off, insects were chirping everywhere, and god knows what small animals were scuttling around in the dry leaves at my feet. But even here, I couldn't stop thinking about what had been keeping me awake, about what had happened at the hospital that afternoon.

(STAND AND WALK A FEW STEPS)

I'm in the outpatient clinic. I've just examined one of our pregnant patients, who's doing well, when I feel a tap on my arm.

(LOOK UP SLIGHTLY TO LEFT, SMILE)

"*Oi Celestino, como você está?*"

"*Oi, Doutora, tudo bem?* Sorry to bother, but I'm worried about those two brothers in the TB ward. I need you to come right away to see them."

(WALK FORWARD, SPEAK TO AUDIENCE)

Celestino's my favorite nurse. He's 18 or 19 years old, tall and thin with dark brown skin and a beaurtiful smile, which always sets the patients at ease. He was a medic during the Angolan civil war, and has great medical skills. He also has excellent medical judgement, so if he's worried, I'm worried.

(WALK BEHIND CHAIR TO STAGE RIGHT)

As we walk to the tuberculosis ward, another big army tent, we put on our protective masks. They fit tightly around our noses and mouths, and are squashed onto our faces by two strong elastic bands. In order for us to breathe, they come out in front in sort of a duckbill shape. For some reason they're pink.

(WALK STAGE LEFT, THEN RIGHT SLOWLY, LOOKING AT BROTHERS)

Inside, the brothers are waiting for us, each sitting on his cot, each with a packed bag next to him. They're in their early twenties, skeletally thin, covered with a sheen of sweat, and panting even though they're just sitting still. They cough a lot, into their own duckbilled masks.

(SIT)

"*O que esta acontesendo?* How can I help?"

(STAND WITH DIFFICULTY, BEND OVER, BREATH FAST, LEFT HAND ON BACK OF CHAIR)

"*Doutora*"

(COUGH, COUGH, COUGH, RIGHT HAND UP, DEEP BREATH)

"We've been here four days now, taking all the medicines and eating as much as we can of the good food, but we're no better! We still have high fevers; we can't sleep because of coughing we're so weak we have to help each other walk to the latrine.

The truth is, *as suas medicinas nâo funcionan pra gente*. We talked it over and we've figured out why. It's because our sickness comes from a spell cast by our uncle after I argued with him about land last month. We need to go back to the village right away, to get the *curandeiro* and the elders to help us break the spell. Otherwise we'll just die here like that old man in the corner bed did yesterday!"

(POINT TWO-HANDED GESTURE)

Four duckbills turn and look at the empty bed, remembering.

(DROP ARMS, PAUSE, WALk FORWARD AND ADDRESS THE AUDIENCE)

But seriously, spells? These two guys dressed like me and Celestino inT-shirts and jeans, articulate and well-spoken, were the last people I expected to talk to me about spells! I'd been to their village: in the market I'd bought a garish Che Guevara T-shirt, and a pirated Michael Jackson cd! I'd watched television in the village cafe: soap operas, sports, and news, from Angola, from all of Africa, from all over the world! Sure, their village was isolated, but they weren't isolated from the world of the 21st century!

I honestly didn't know what to say to them. Celestino saved me.

(PICK UP CHAIR AND POSITION IT FACING SLIGHTLY TO RIGHT, SIT, LEAN BACK, SMILE)

"My friends... let me tell you a story. Just three months ago my mother brought my younger brother here, from our village. She hadn't even told me he was sick! When I saw him for the first time...

(LEAN FORWARD, HANDS ON KNEES, LOOK DOWN, SHAKE HEAD)

...I thought he was going to die right in front of me! He was thinner than you are, coughing blood, weak. We brought him to this tent. For the first five days I took him water, helped him take his pills, fed him, carried him to the latrine, and little by little he was coughing less, his fevers were going down, and he started eating. Three more weeks and he was strong enough to go home and continue the pills there.

Now when people come from there they tell me he's walking from our house to the market every day! He's getting fat!

(BIG LAUGH, PAUSE, HAND OVER HEART)

I know... If he'd gone home after just a few days, stopping the treatment, right now...he would be dead."

(STAND, LEFT HAND ON CHAIR BACK, HOARSE VOICE)

"Well that just shows that his sickness wasn't caused by a spell, like ours was. No wonder he got well. Look. (GASP) Brother!!

(DROP TO KNEES, COUGH REPEATEDLY, UNCONTROLLABLY, THEN PULL UP MASK, COUGH, HAWK, SPIT, PULL MASK DOWN, START DIGGING)

The younger brother hawks up a thick wad of green phlegm, covered with red blood, then starts digging up the tent floor - which is dirt of course - he piles dirt over the mess till it's completely covered, then tamps it down till it hardly shows.

(LOOK DOWN AT MESS)

Omigod, this must be what they all do!

(PAUSE)

Before my eyes, the tent floor turns into a collection of covered-over messes of green, bloody phlegm.

(LOOK AT AUDIENCE)

Actually that's an effective method of infection control. It starves the TB germs of air, they die, and they can't infect anyone else. We help the younger brother back up onto his cot.

(HAND HIM A CLOTH FROM MY BACK POCKET)

"Here, wipe your face."

(RIGHT HAND ON HIS SHOULDER)

"You ok?"

(SIT, LOOK AT OLDER BROTHER)

"I understand what you're saying. I've heard about these spells, and when I think about them I feel scared too. But look at me - I'm not a new doctor, I'm not a young doctor. I've treated many people with tuberculosis. I know this sickness. I know these medicines. And right now, in this part of Angola, where we're just starting to see more cases, they are working. They will make you better.

(STAND)

So let me offer you this: you stay three more days, taking the medicines and eating the good food. If you're no better at all on the fourth day, I will personally take our jeep and drive you six hours to the big hospital in Malange City. We can get X-rays there, and blood tests, and other doctors can examine you. What do you say, just three more days?

(STAND BREATHLESS, ONE HAND ON HIP)

"Let me offer you this, *Doutora*! We stay here three more days, and if we're no better on the fourth day you take the jeep and drive us to our village, to break the spell. If that doesn't work, then we'll come back here and you can drive us to your big hospital."

(WALK FORWARD, TALK TO AUDIENCE)

Of course I'll take the three days! I'll lose them completely if I don't.

(STAND BEHIND CHAIR, HANDS ON CHAIR, SPEAK TO AUDIENCE)

I had to go out of the village for meetings, for the next few days. Whenever I had time alone, I thought about this case. I began second-guessing myself: why had I asked them to stay only three more days? Would that be enough time for them to actually start to feel better? What if I had the wrong doses of the medications? Or the wrong medications in the first place? What if they didn't have TB? I even caught myself wondering if their uncle really had cast a spell on them...

(WALK AROUND CHAIR, FORWARD)

The stakes were high. Not just their lives were at risk, but those of their family members and neighbors, whom they would likely infect if they stopped treatment. If they left the hospital, would there be a mass exodus of TB patients? Would the community at large lose confidence in the TB program? If it crumbled, would Angola kick Doctors Without Borders out of the country? Would I be kicked out of Doctors Without Borders?

(WALK TO THE OTHER SIDE OF THE STAGE)

The morning of the fourth day I walked up to the hospital, dreading what I would find: two corpses? two empty beds? An empty TB tent? I peered around the doorjamb of our morning meeting room, searching for Celestino.

(WALK SLOWLY, ARMS OUT SMILING)

(SPEAKING SLOWLY)

"*Doutora* Barbara...bem vindo! The brothers haven't coughed up one drop of blood since our conversation, and last night they slept better than they have in months! They're going to stay!"

Without thinking I threw my arms around him. We both jumped back. All the nurses were laughing. I was so relieved, I was shaking. I had to take a moment to gather myself.

(TURN AROUND SLOWLY, THEN LOOK AT WRISTWATCH)

"Well, time for morning rounds. Let's go!"

Picture This

Picture this: a long, straight, black paved road, with nothing but dry, brown, packed earth on both sides, stretching as far as the eye can see. Temperature around 102-104 F, with a dry wind blowing.

I'm driving a white van, sitting in the front seat with the only two passengers, a boy of 13 and his father. Both are dressed in long, white gowns -jellabiyas- with white skull caps. The boy also has on a blue, open vest which comes down to hip level.

I'm transporting them back from a visit to the hospital in Gedaref, the city one hour away from our town of Showak, Sudan. I'd taken him there to see if the psychiatrist could do anything for his florid psychosis, which had begun several days earlier as he began to recover from a bout of cerebral malaria. He'd had a seizure, common in cerebral malaria, which we had stopped with IV Valium, but he had been incoherent, sobbing and shouting, ever since.

His fever was gone and he'd completed his course of Chloroquin for the malaria, but his mental status had not returned to normal. He was disturbing the many other patients in his ward, who were also recovering from malaria, and was driving the health workers crazy.

In the big hospital in Gedaref the psychiatrist had given him an injection of the antipsychotic Haldol, which had calmed him. He recommended continuing the drug until the boy remained calm for 12 hours after the last dose. I asked about side effects, and the doc just said to use Benadryl or Valium if any developed.

So as we're driving along, I glance over at the boy and see that his mouth is gaping open, wide. His father is talking to him, pushing up on his lower jaw, trying to get him to close it. His jaw is frozen in this position (think the painting "The Scream"), and I see that his fingers are cramped and stiff. Sure enough, he's having a dystonic reaction to the Haldol (severe cramping of all his muscles), an unfortunately all-too-common risk with use of antipsychotics.

Luckily, the health worker who had come with us to the hospital had put a syringe with 10 ml of Valium into my hand as the van he was in took off ahead of us back to Showak. Did he foresee this situation? I asked him later and he said it was always good to have some Valium on hand, especially with a passenger who had just gotten over cerebral malaria, which is sometimes complicated by seizures.

So I pulled off as best I could (no shoulders) to the side of the two-lane highway, asked the father to get out of the passenger seat, turned the boy so he was sitting in that seat facing the now open door (he's stiff as a board by this time with copious amounts of saliva dripping from his wide open mouth). I pantomimed to the father that he should wrap his hands tightly around the upper left arm of the boy to make the vein just below the elbow stand out. I wiped the area quickly with an alcohol swab (never leave home without one) and plunged the needle of the syringe into the vein being kept open by his human tourniquet (the father). I blasted in 10 mg of Valium.

I'm thinking, "Oh god, his father's watching all this; what if it doesn't work?" I had no other medications or medical supplies with me.

The boy immediately began to relax, closed his mouth, and wiped off his face. As I climbed back into the van I looked around at the hot, bleak landscape and said to myself, "No one will ever believe this!"

We poured him back into position between us and I drove more quickly than I should've back to our clinic in Showak. He remained relaxed and I gave him a whopping injection of Benadryl as soon as we got there.

Unfortunately, as soon as the Haldol, Valium and Benadryl wore off, he was back to screaming and crying. The next day the health workers convinced me to let our driver take him and his father to the mental hospital a few days away. I knew I had nothing more to offer him, but I had no idea what this mental hospital was like.

Happy Ending: several weeks later he and his father showed up at our clinic, to say hello and thank me. They were on their way home from the mental hospital. The boy was calm, smiling, appreciative, completely normal! His father said he didn't know what the doctors had given him, but he wasn't sent home with any medications. I suspect they had treated him with electroconvulsive therapy ("shock treatments") but I'll never know for sure...

Angry Man

It was a busy afternoon in the Delek Tibetan Hospital in Dharamsala, India. I was working in the small emergency room, checking a patient who'd just finished an asthma breathing treatment, when I heard loud voices. A burly young Tibetan man rushed in holding his three year old son in his arms. A rag was wrapped tightly around the child's left hand. The father was quite agitated, and there was a strong smell of alcohol on his breath. The child was wailing. A visibly worried, quiet woman followed behind them. I turned the asthma patient over to a colleague and asked the father what was wrong. He said his son's finger had almost been cut off, and angrily yelled at his wife that it was her fault. He kept up an angry barrage of words, mostly in Tibetan, some in broken English, as I unwrapped the child's hand. I asked him to lower his voice but he didn't. Of course a crowd was gathering: other patients, their family members, and staff.

When the hand was exposed, I saw that the little finger had been deeply cut just above the last joint, and was oozing blood, but that it was by no means cut off and that a repair would be possible. Upon seeing it the father again began yelling at his wife, and even went so far as to kick at her legs. At that point I asked one of the nurses to get the hospital administrator, to come help defuse the situation. I placed a clean gauze around the finger and had the mother hold gentle pressure on it to stop the bleeding. The administrator soon arrived and it turned out he knew the father, which helped matters. I asked him to explain to the father that I could sew the finger back together, but that if he didn't quiet down and show some respect to the hospital staff and to his wife, I would not help his child. A number of onlookers chimed in, insisting that the man shut up and sit down (as I later learned through a translator). So Dad was led off by the administrator for a cup of tea, and I could begin my work.

Then I had to convince the nurse on duty that I actually could sew the finger back on. My experience as an emergency physician made me confident that I could, and I knew that the alternative, sending the child to the Indian government hospital a half hour's drive away, which had a surgeon, would be no guarantee of better treatment. I'd seen their Casualty (Emergency) department and it was less well-stocked than ours. I'd also taken critical patients there and waited an agonizingly long time for any doctor to appear.

These parents didn't speak Hindi, and so would have a difficult time negotiating that system, especially with the father hostile and inebriated.

I just smiled at the nurse, told her I understood that she didn't know me very well and asked her to trust me, that I'd had a lot of experience sewing up little fingers. I said I knew with her expertise and help we'd be able to do it together. She looked doubtful. "We always transfer out bad cuts," but she started to get out the supplies. Mom stayed with the child, who'd calmed down by then.

We started out by giving the child a shot of Ketamine, which put him into a "twilight sleep." Then I could inject a numbing medicine into the injured finger itself and clean it well without causing further pain. Close inspection showed that the fleshy tip of the finger beyond the cut had slipped off the bone (which wasn't broken), and so the end of the finger appeared to be dangling. But actually the cut only went halfway across the finger, and none of the flesh or skin was missing.

I cleaned the injured parts well, pulled the flesh into position over the bone, and stitched it into place. I knew the fingertip might remain numb for months or longer, but otherwise the finger should return to normal. Of course there are always possibilities of infection or lack of circulation causing the entire end of the finger to blacken and fall off... These visions were definitely in the back of my mind as I worked. A bad outcome would've not only threatened the child's well-being, but also the community's trust in the hospital and in the volunteer doctors, not to mention the staff's confidence in me. Medicine is full of risks.

Luckily, the fingertip remained viable. I saw the patient in follow-up every three or four days - I was that worried about a possible adverse outcome. No one was happier than I to see the little pink finger emerge after ten days of antibiotics and the final removal of the stitches.

Dad accompanied his son to each visit and was all smiles and appreciation, though always with a faint aroma of alcohol about his person. Alcoholism is not common among the Tibetans in Dharamsala, but he was a well-known drinker and wife-abuser. We were able to refer him to the psychiatrist who worked with the hospital, as well as to the Tibetan staff of the local drug and alcohol abuse program, but he never once even said he thought he should stop drinking. "It's my habit, what can I do?" he'd ask with a smile. On each visit he was roundly and loudly lectured by the sharp-tongued nurses about his drinking.

His wife never came with him. I asked the nurses about her...they said they couldn't understand why she stayed with him, or why she'd married him in the first place. They weren't very sympathetic. (some things are universal). I asked if there was a support group to which we could refer her and one of the nurses agreed to look into it. With the busyness of the hospital the case soon faded into the background, but remains clear in my memory, with all its surgical and social ramifications.

A Close Call

Chinzum came running down the hallway toward me. In her long nurse's uniform, with the striped apron that signified that she was married, she shouted,

"*Dotte-la*, you speak French, don't you?"

Chinzum never ran, so I knew it must really be an emergency. I followed the cloud of blue cotton down the hall.

The scene in the entryway: a tall, muscular blond man, who looked to be in his mid-twenties, was being led into the hospital by two young women, one holding each hand.

"*Mais, lâchez-moi, lâchez-moi!*" He struggled as the girls spoke loudly to him in French. Chinzum and two other nurses were trying English:

"What's wrong sir? Are you sick?" then arguing with each other in Tibetan.

"*Tashi tashi delek, tashi delek!*" It was a real Tower of Babel.

Everything went quiet as I entered the room.

The man was frowning, trying to get his hands free, looking around wildly, but not making eye contact with anyone. His hair was messed up, he kept clenching his fists, he was breathing fast, sweating. His eyes were dilated.

"OK, OK, *bonjour, bienvenue, je m'appele Barbara*." I let my white coat slide to the floor as I sat on the couch. "Please, sit down. Would you like a cup of tea?" Chinzum was way ahead of me; she'd already gestured to the *chai wallah* (Sara and I privately referred to him as the tea dude), who came every morning at 10:30, and was right on time. Pretty soon I and the three Europeans were sipping cups of hot, sweet, milky tea.

The girls had found Philippe, which turned out to be his name, pacing and speaking loudly in French to no one in particular when they came out of a store, so they'd hailed a taxi and brought him to our hospital. They knew only his name. I thanked them for helping a stranger in need, though as they left I was thinking, "Oh god, why did they bring him here? Now I have to figure out what to do with him!"

I was really worried about this man. Ten years in the ER had shown me that a young man who acts like this is either mentally ill and having a psychotic break, on meth or cocaine, or withdrawing from an alcohol binge. Either way,

I knew he could go off at any moment, could hurt himself or someone else. As if to illustrate, he abruptly got up, teacup shattering on the floor, and started pacing around the entryway. Chinzum and I guided him out onto the sun porch, where a young patient, his leg swathed in bandages, was strumming his guitar. I gestured him over.

"Could you play over here please, for our new friend?" ...music to soothe the savage beast.

He seemed to tune into the music. I asked him how long he'd been in India. He looked down, mumbled,

"*Arrivé ce matin*" He'd arrived that morning.

"Why did you come right away to Dharamsala?"

He pulled out a slip of paper on which was written a French woman's name, and a phone number. Chinzum immediately whisked it out of his hand.

"I'll call the number." I knew she was worried. The medical director was out of town, so she as the nurse in charge, and I as the doctor on duty, would have to jointly decide what to do.

Philippe sat down again and a new cup of tea was brought. Chinzum came back and said the number was of a friend of his family, Sylvie, who was on her way to the hospital. I translated into French, and he actually smiled.

"Ah, Sylvie."

So this small, short-haired Swiss woman arrived,

"*Bonjour, bonjour, je suis Sylvie. Philippe!*" (kiss kiss) They sat down and started chatting in French. Philippe visibly relaxed. I let the young Tibetan patient stop playing; he got a cup of tea too. I whispered to Chinzum to prepare a syringe with 10 mg of Valium.

Philippe was starting to look nervous again. The guitarist saw this and started to play. Sylvie's phone rang; it was Philippe's sister in Switzerland, returning her call. She listened for a while, then put Philippe on the line. While he talked with his sister, Sylvie told me and Chinzum that he had bipolar disorder, and had left his medications at home, thinking he wouldn't need them in India. The sister had arranged through the Swiss National Health Service to send an ambulance with a psychiatrist from New Delhi to Dharamsala to pick up Philippe early the next morning and take him to a psychiatric hospital especially for acutely mentally ill tourists. (Who knew they were so common?!) He'd be medicated and stabilized in Delhi and flown back to Switzerland. A solution!

Suddenly Philippe got up, dropped the phone, pulled a large handkerchief from his back pocket, and began rapidly cleaning the couch they'd been sitting in. He moved onto a chair, then started working on the windows. I'd seen a lot of acute psychosis, I knew he was trying to calm himself. But a chair could quickly become a weapon. I really needed to sedate him. I knew that would commit us to keeping him in the hospital, but now it would only be till the next morning.

Two nurses were looking in from the doorway to the sunroom. Taking advantage of the fact that Philippe knew no English, I asked one of them to run upstairs to Administration and bring down four men, right away. "Tell them it's an emergency!" Philippe kept cleaning. When the men were assembled, I called out their names one by one, assigning each to a limb.

"Wagmo, right arm, Tenzin left arm, Tsering right leg, Namgyal left leg." Chinzum passed me the syringe which I put in my back pocket. Sylvie sat back on the couch and beckoned to Philippe to join her there.

You'd have thought we'd choreographed it. The men and I walked quickly but nonchalantly toward Philippe. Sylvie started singing what sounded like a children's song, which briefly distracted him. I shouted at the others to come in and grab their assigned limbs, and pull him onto the couch. It all happened so fast - the others grabbed his arms and legs; as he went down onto the couch Chinzum turned him onto his back and put her arms under his head; I plunged the needle into a large vein in his right arm, and steadily pushed 10 mg of valium directly into his blood stream. I heard Sylvie singing throughout the whole thing. Peace at last; his eyes closed and he was asleep. We carried him to one of the empty hospital beds in the men's ward. His color was good, he was breathing easily, heartbeat was normal.

After thanking everyone for helping me, I turned to Chinzum. I was relieved, proud, elated - he was sedated, no one had been hurt, only a teacup had been broken! I smiled at her in relief, but she didn't smile back. She wouldn't even meet my eyes. I was stunned, hurt, and then got mad - what was that all about? I'd averted a possible crisis, staved off chaos, and she wouldn't share it with me? Well if that was what she wanted it, so be it.

"Chinzum, please draw up one syringe of 50 mg of Benadryl, and another with 5 mg of Haldol." I spoke firmly, no smile. "Be sure to label each one as soon as you fill it."

"OK *Dotte-la*." She walked to the medication room.

When she handed me the syringes, I injected Philippe with the additional drugs intramuscularly. They would last about six hours.

Still looking down, Chinzum said,

"We usually just call the police when we get a patient like this, especially if it's a tourist or an Indian. They handcuff them and take them to the big Regional hospital and drop them off."

"But I knew we could handle him here, and take good care of him; and we had some empty beds."

"We don't usually spend so much time and energy on them."

"Let's put him in the private room for tonight. I'll stay and sleep right outside it myself, and medicate him through the night if he needs it."

She said nothing.

So I just let it go.

"If you really think we should call the ambulance, go ahead. I can't stop you. You have to do what you think is right."

She just looked at her wristwatch.

"My shift is over." She turned and left the hospital. The nurse coming on duty and I rolled Philippe into the private room.

As I ate dinner that evening, I reflected on the whole incident. It dawned on me that it had been a power struggle, but I didn't feel good about "winning" it. I had been so focused on the immediate problem this patient presented, and so elated that my treatment had worked, that I hadn't considered the big picture. I was just there temporarily, for six months, because they didn't have enough doctors. They appreciated us volunteers, but also resented us as outsiders, especially if they felt that we pushed them around. I remembered the first baby I'd delivered there: just as it was crowning, Chinzum had said,

"You have to cut now, *Dotte-la*; quick, cut!" I knew the baby was small enough that it wouldn't need the extra room an episiotomy would give, and simply didn't do it.

"Chinzum, all mothers don't need to be cut." She'd looked shocked, then angry, but never said a word. Mother and baby were fine.

Another time we'd clashed was when an Indian woman brought her elderly father to the hospital, with symptoms of a stroke in progress. As I examined him, I noted his finger stumps; a sign of leprosy. His daughter saw me looking, and immediately told me he'd been treated years ago at the nearby leprosarium. I knew his leprosy was "burned out", and therefore not contagious (I'd been reading up on leprosy, and had visited the nearby leprosarium just the week before.) I wanted to admit him, lower his blood pressure with medications, and start physical therapy. But Chinzum was adamant that if we admitted a leper, the Tibetans would stop coming to the hospital. I was dismayed that the Tibetan medical professionals at the hospital, who'd all been born in India, knew so little about the natural course of the disease. I lost that battle; the whole staff was arrayed against me. I could see that the medical director didn't want to side with me, the foreigner, against his local staff.

Tibetans are refugees in India, not Indian citizens, and feel all the insecurity every refugee feels. They don't care that western volunteers and tourists respect Tibetan Bhuddism and admire the Dalai Lama; they're just trying to survive, raise their families, not rock the boat.

I didn't sleep much that night; I had to get up and medicate Philippe twice. At 7 AM the Delhi ambulance was there. I compared notes with the psychiatrist who assured me my total dose of 30 mg of Haldol was not unusual in cases of acute psychosis like this one, especially in a young healthy man. He congratulated me on my handling of the case.

But Chinzum never forgave me.

We barely saw each other after that; I noticed she was never assigned to assist me.

I'm still not sure I did the right thing, though I felt good when Sylvie and I had lunch together a couple of weeks later. She showed me a letter from Philippe - lucid and logical - saying he was back on his meds, doing well, working, studying.... and that he couldn't thank all of us enough.

Broken Heart

The 18 month old girl lay in her mother's arms, feverish, rigid, heart racing. Her eyes were locked in a gaze to one side, her mouth open and dry. She had been admitted to the ward the night before by the health worker on call, who had correctly assessed her condition as grave and had called her parents to sit with her, but who had incorrectly treated her with only a penicillin shot and a Tylenol suppository.

The staff of our health center, in this dusty town in remote northern Sudan, brought me to see the infant as soon as I arrived for morning rounds. A brief exam convinced me she had meningitis.

Stifling my irritation at her substandard care, I silently reminded myself that these health workers were doing a hard job with minimal training, not to mention having to struggle with my language as I barely spoke theirs. So I smiled after my frown, but told them this was an urgent case.

I ordered an intravenous line to be started, through which 500 mg of our precious stock of the antibiotic ceftriaxone would be administered, along with water containing sugar and salt, to keep the parched child alive. I added the steroid dexamethasone and an injection of an additional antibiotic, streptomycin, in case TB germs were present.

Mother and father were instructed to wet the towels they'd brought at the courtyard faucet, and place them on her head and abdomen. They fanned her continuously to break her fever. If she showed signs of surviving I'd do a spinal tap and draw lab tests later in the day.

As the health workers hurried to carry out these orders, I took a deep breath and surveyed the thatch-roofed circular hut or *tookel* which served as our Pediatrics ward. Six beds lined the walls, each containing a small figure surrounded by family members. These family members provided all food and bedding for the patients, and even administered some of their oral medicines. Natural light streamed in through the single door and through the windows cut every two to three feet in the wall.

Before I could round on the other patients, an emaciated three year old boy was rushed in, burning with fever, unconscious, with extremely pale gums, palms, and nails. It being malaria season, with heavy rains every afternoon, his diagnosis was almost certainly coma due to falciparum malaria, complicated by malnutrition and severe anemia.

We laid him on the dirt floor on blankets his parents had brought. Physical exam showed him to be dehydrated, with dry mouth and skin. He had an enlarged spleen on the left side of his abdomen, confirming the diagnosis of malaria. Again postponing lab tests, I ordered an intravenous line to be placed for the treatment of Quinine mixed with sugar-containing water. A Tylenol suppository was inserted and I set his mother to placing wet towels on his little body and fanning him. I pulled his father aside to discuss the need for a volunteer blood donor from the family. But as we were talking his wife suddenly screamed and the whole family began to wail. The boy had died before the IV could even be inserted.

I rushed to the bedside, but the relatives pushed me aside. I stood back as they cried and prayed over the child, having learned that while sickness might be my domain, death was theirs.

I sadly turned away to tend to a six year old girl, already on IV Quinine, who unbelievably went into a seizure just at that moment. The health worker who'd earlier started the IV on the girl with meningitis ran over at my shout and began to give IV Valium to stop the convulsion while I lifted the child's chin to open the airway and held her tongue down with the double tongue depressor, which was taped to each bedstead. As her shaking slowed and then stopped, and the three year old's family carried his body away, silence fell in the *tookel*. The unstated question hung in the air, "Will this happen to my child?"

I shakily finished rounds, then stepped outside. I leaned against a pole holding up the thatched roof of the porch and said aloud,

"I've got to get out of here before my heart breaks." No one near me spoke English... the words were for me alone.

www.ingramcontent.com/pod-product-compliance
Lightning Source LLC
LaVergne TN
LVRC082252220926
848486LV00046B/394

* 9 7 9 8 2 9 5 4 1 8 9 4 5 *